BREAKING FREE: OVERCOMING THE GRIP OF DRUG ADDICTION

A COMPREHENSIVE GUIDE TO RECLAIMING YOUR LIFE AND EMBRACING RECOVERY

Robert Brooks

TABLE OF CONTENT

INTRODUCTION

In the shadows cast by the gripping force of drug addiction, there exists a journey toward liberation. This comprehensive guide, "Breaking Free: Overcoming the Grip of Drug Addiction," invites you to embark on a transformative exploration. In the intricate tapestry of recovery, we navigate the complexities of addiction, weaving a narrative that illuminates both the shadows and the light that awaits beyond.

Unveiling the Journey Addiction

like a silent conductor orchestrating a symphony of challenges, often masks itself in the subtleties of everyday life. This guide begins by unveiling the layers of addiction, peeling back the intricate patterns that bind individuals to its grasp. We delve into the roots, exploring the psychological, social, and biological facets that contribute to the allure of substances. "Breaking Free" is not just a guide; it is a revelation, a mirror held up to the complexities of addiction, allowing you to recognize the chains that have taken hold.

The Promise of Recovery

Amidst the exploration of addiction's depths, the guide carries a promise—a promise of recovery, resilience, and the reclamation of life. We confront the stigma that often shrouds those navigating the path to recovery. Each page is a step toward dispelling myths and fostering understanding. This introduction lays the foundation for the transformative journey that lies ahead—a journey that goes beyond the mere cessation of substance use.

Comprehensive Guidance
The subtitle, "A Comprehensive Guide to Reclaiming Your Life and Embracing Recovery," encapsulates the essence of our endeavour. This is not merely a roadmap; it is a comprehensive companion. Each chapter unfolds as a crucial piece of the puzzle, offering insights into the science of addiction, strategies for breaking free, and the intricate process of rebuilding a life once ensnared by substances.

Invitation to the Reader

As you immerse yourself in "Breaking Free," consider this not just a guide but an invitation—an invitation to self-discovery, resilience, and the pursuit of a sober existence. Whether you are on the brink of acknowledging a struggle with addiction or supporting someone on this journey, this guide seeks to empower and inform.

Continuation to Series 1

The introduction serves as the gateway to a five-part series, each segment carefully crafted to address specific facets of the recovery journey. It is not merely a prelude; it is a call to action. We embark on Series 1, "Foundations of Understanding," where we unravel the intricacies of addiction, laying the groundwork for the practical steps that follow.

In the following pages, we explore the hidden triggers, the impact on brain chemistry, and the societal influences that shape the narrative of addiction. As we conclude Series 1, the transition seamlessly unfolds into Series 2, promising a journey from awareness to action.

"Breaking Free" is not just a guide; it is an odyssey—one that transcends the boundaries of addiction, leading toward the promise of a life reclaimed. So, let the journey begin, for within these pages lies the power to break free and embrace the boundless possibilities of recovery.

Chapter 1: Introduction to Addiction

In the labyrinth of human experience, addiction emerges as a formidable force, transcending the boundaries of choice and behaviour. This chapter serves as an inaugural step into the profound journey of "Unmasking Addiction," aiming to unravel the layers that cloak this complex phenomenon.

The Pervasive Nature of Addiction

Addiction, often misconstrued as a mere lapse in judgement or a series of poor decisions, reveals itself to be a nuanced interplay of factors. It transcends the realm of conscious choices, delving into the intricate tapestry of biology, psychology, and societal influences. This introduction invites readers to set aside preconceived notions, urging them to embrace a holistic perspective that acknowledges addiction's pervasive nature.

Beyond Behaviour: Understanding the Roots

To unmask addiction, one must first recognize it as more than a surface-level behaviour. It is an intricate dance of neurochemistry, a response to psychological needs, and a reflection of societal dynamics. As we embark on this exploration, it becomes clear that addiction is a symptom, not just a problem. The introduction lays the groundwork for understanding addiction as a manifestation of deeper challenges, urging readers to look beyond the surface.

The Cycle of Vulnerability

Acknowledging the cyclical nature of addiction is crucial to comprehending its relentless grip. The introductory chapter unfolds the stages of addiction, from the initial encounter with substances to the compounding consequences. By dissecting this cycle, readers gain insight into the vulnerabilities that pave the way for addiction's progression. It is a journey marked by susceptibility, and understanding these stages is the key to breaking free.

The Lens of Compassion

In approaching addiction, the chapter emphasizes the importance of adopting a lens of compassion. It calls upon readers to recognize the individuals grappling with addiction not as mere statistics or labels but as complex human beings navigating a challenging path. By fostering empathy, the introduction sets the tone for dismantling judgement and embracing a collective responsibility in addressing addiction as a societal concern.

From Stigma to Understanding

Society's perception of addiction often veers into the realm of stigma, hindering open discourse and impeding the path to recovery. This chapter challenges societal norms, unravelling the impact of judgement and misrepresentation. By shedding light on the stigma surrounding addiction, readers are encouraged to re-evaluate their perspectives and contribute to a more supportive and understanding environment.

The Promise of Knowledge

As the introduction unfolds, it carries with it a promise—the promise of knowledge as a catalyst for change. It asserts that by understanding the intricate nature of addiction, individuals can empower themselves to break free from its chains. This promise forms the foundation upon which the subsequent chapters will build, guiding readers toward a comprehensive understanding that transcends stereotypes and misconceptions.

Inviting Reflection

The chapter concludes by inviting readers to reflect on their own perceptions of addiction. It challenges preconceived notions, prompting a journey of self-discovery. Through this introspection, readers are encouraged to set aside biases and engage with the forthcoming content with an open mind—a mind ready to absorb the complexities of addiction and, in doing so, contribute to the collective effort of breaking free.

Conclusion of Chapter 1:

As readers close the inaugural chapter, the introduction to addiction lingers as a call to awareness. The curtain has been drawn back, revealing the intricate dance of factors that shape the narrative of addiction. This chapter is not a conclusion but a commencement—a gateway into the exploration of deeper layers in the chapters that follow. In recognizing addiction's multifaceted nature, readers embark on a transformative journey, armed with the knowledge that understanding is the first step toward breaking free from the chains that bind.

Chapter 2: The Cycle of Addiction

In the intricate tapestry of addiction, understanding its cyclical nature is fundamental to unravelling the chains that bind individuals. Chapter 2, "The Cycle of Addiction," delves into the stages and patterns that define this relentless journey, shedding light on the nuances that perpetuate the struggle.

The Initial Encounter: Allure and Escapism

At the genesis of the addiction cycle lies the initial encounter—a moment where substances weave their allure. Whether driven by curiosity, peer influence, or a quest for escape, individuals take their first steps into the intricate web of addiction. This chapter scrutinizes this initial phase, exploring the factors that contribute to the allure and the temporary relief it promises.

Escalation: The Unfolding Drama

From the initial encounter, the cycle escalates as individuals grapple with escalating consequences. What begins as a seemingly innocuous experiment transforms into a coping mechanism, providing solace in the face of life's challenges. Chapter 2 delves into the unfolding drama, dissecting the progression from occasional use to regular patterns and the compounding impact on physical and mental well-being.

Compounding Consequences: The Ties That Bind

As the cycle advances, the consequences of addiction become increasingly entwined with daily life. Employment, relationships, and overall well-being are jeopardized. This chapter scrutinizes the compounding consequences, unravelling the intricate ties that bind individuals to their addictive behaviours. It explores the ways in which the cycle tightens its grip, making breaking free a formidable challenge.

The Illusion of Control: Denial and Rationalization

A hallmark of the addiction cycle is the illusion of control. Chapter 2 dives into the psychological mechanisms of denial and rationalization that individuals employ to convince themselves that they maintain control over their substance use. By dissecting this aspect, the chapter exposes the deceptive nature of addiction, where individuals convince themselves that they are immune to its grasp.

Repercussions on Relationships: Strained Bonds

The cycle of addiction extends its tendrils to the fabric of relationships. Strained bonds, shattered trust, and emotional turmoil become prevalent as individuals navigate the repercussions of their addiction. This chapter sheds light on the impact of addiction on interpersonal connections, emphasizing the collateral damage that extends far beyond the individual.

Seeking Relief: The Cycle Reinforced

As the consequences mount, the addictive cycle reinforces itself through a perpetual quest for relief. Individuals caught in this cycle use substances not only for pleasure but as a means to escape the mounting challenges. Chapter 2 explores the paradoxical nature of seeking relief in the very source of distress, perpetuating the cycle and deepening the chains of addiction.

Intervention Points: Breaking the Cycle

Amidst the seemingly relentless cycle, there exist intervention points—opportunities to disrupt the patterns and initiate change. This chapter highlights these pivotal moments, encouraging readers to recognize the potential for intervention in their own journeys or in supporting others. Whether through personal insight, external assistance, or a combination of both, breaking the cycle begins with acknowledging the existence of these critical junctures.

The Impact on Mental Health: A Vicious Interplay

The cycle of addiction intricately intertwines with mental health. Chapter 2 navigates the complex interplay, examining how addiction exacerbates existing mental health challenges and often gives rise to new ones. By understanding this vicious interplay, readers gain insights into the importance of holistic approaches to recovery that address both substance use and mental well-being.

Conclusion of Chapter 2:

As readers conclude the exploration of "The Cycle of Addiction," they are left with a profound understanding of the intricate dance that ensnares individuals in addiction's grasp. This chapter is not merely an analysis of behaviour; it is an invitation to reflect on personal experiences and recognize the various entry points for breaking free. As the journey unfolds, the interplay between allure, consequences, and seeking relief serves as a roadmap—a guide toward intervention and the possibility of reclaiming one's life from the cyclical chains of addiction.

Chapter 3: Hidden Triggers: Unravelling Influences

In the intricate landscape of addiction, the origins and triggers that propel individuals into the cycle of substance use often lie concealed beneath the surface. Chapter 3, "Hidden Triggers: Unravelling Influences," embarks on a journey to expose these subtle forces, providing a nuanced understanding of the influences that contribute to the initiation and perpetuation of addiction.

The Veiled Catalysts

The chapter begins by acknowledging that addiction seldom arises in isolation. Rather, it is often influenced by an array of hidden triggers that shape an individual's relationship with substances. From childhood experiences and trauma to environmental stresses, these triggers are the subtle catalysts that set the stage for the allure of substances.

Psychological Undercurrents: Coping and Escapism

Psychological triggers play a pivotal role in the initiation of substance use. Chapter 3 delves into the undercurrents of the human psyche, exploring how individuals turn to substances as coping mechanisms or means of escape. By unravelling the intricacies of these psychological triggers, readers gain insight into the emotional landscapes that contribute to the allure of addiction.

Social Influences: The Power of Peer Dynamics
The influence of social circles and peer dynamics cannot be underestimated. This chapter scrutinizes the impact of social influences on substance use, illuminating how individuals may be drawn into the cycle through peer pressure, societal norms, or a desire for social acceptance. By understanding these external forces, readers are equipped to navigate the social complexities that can contribute to hidden triggers.

Environmental Factors: Setting the Stage

Environments, both familial and societal, play a crucial role in shaping an individual's relationship with substances. Chapter 3 explores the environmental factors that set the stage for hidden triggers, from family dynamics and socio-economic conditions to cultural influences. Recognizing the profound impact of these environments is essential for understanding the roots of addiction.

Trauma and Unresolved Pain: Lingering Shadows

Unresolved trauma and emotional pain often cast lingering shadows that drive individuals toward substance use. This chapter delves into the connection between trauma and addiction, unrevealing how past experiences can become hidden triggers. By shining a light on these shadows, readers are encouraged to acknowledge and address the underlying pain that may fuel addictive behaviours.

Routine and Rituals: Unconscious Patterns

The insidious nature of addiction often manifests in routine and rituals. Chapter 3 investigates how seemingly mundane aspects of daily life can become hidden triggers, perpetuating the cycle of substance use. By examining these unconscious patterns, readers gain insight into the ways in which behaviour become deeply ingrained and contribute to the allure of substances.

Media and Cultural Influences: Shaping Perceptions

In the modern age, media and cultural influences exert a significant impact on individuals' perceptions of substance use. This chapter navigates the role of media portrayals, societal norms, and cultural expectations in shaping hidden triggers. By recognizing these external influences, readers can critically assess the narratives surrounding substances and their impact on personal choices.

Personal Narratives: Breaking the Silence

Intertwined with hidden triggers are personal narratives—individual stories that shape one's relationship with substances. Chapter 3 encourages readers to explore their own narratives and the stories of those affected by addiction. By breaking the silence surrounding personal experiences, individuals can gain a deeper understanding of the hidden triggers that have influenced their journey.

Conclusion of Chapter 3:

As readers conclude their exploration of "Hidden Triggers: Unrevealing Influences," they carry with them a heightened awareness of the diverse forces that contribute to addiction's allure. This chapter is not just an analysis of external influences; it is an invitation to introspection—a call to unearth and understand the hidden triggers that may be shaping individual journeys. Armed with this knowledge, readers are better equipped to navigate the complexities of addiction and, in doing so, inch closer to breaking free from the chains that bind.

Chapter 4: The Neurobiology of Addiction

In the intricate dance between the mind and substances, the neurobiology of addiction emerges as a profound force shaping the trajectory of dependence. Chapter 4, "The Neurobiology of Addiction," delves into the intricacies of brain chemistry, neural pathways, and the physiological underpinnings that contribute to the allure and grip of substances.

The Dopamine Reward System: A Pleasure-Seeking Mechanism

At the heart of the neurobiology of addiction lies the dopamine reward system—an ancient mechanism designed to reinforce behaviour essential for survival. Chapter 4 unravels the role of dopamine in the brain, explaining how substances hijack this system, flooding the brain with artificial pleasure signals. This process creates a powerful reinforcement loop, compelling individuals to seek the pleasurable sensations associated with substance use.

Neuroplasticity: Rewiring the Brain

The brain's remarkable ability to adapt, known as neuroplasticity, comes into play in addiction. This chapter explores how repeated substance use alters the structure and function of the brain, creating enduring changes in neural pathways.

Neuroplasticity not only reinforces addictive behaviours but also makes breaking free a formidable challenge, as the brain becomes wired to prioritize substance-related rewards.

Reward Deficiency Syndrome: Craving for Balance

In some cases, individuals may experience a phenomenon known as Reward Deficiency Syndrome (RDS), where the brain's reward system is inherently deficient. Chapter 4 delves into how RDS can contribute to a heightened vulnerability to addiction, as individuals seek substances to compensate for a perceived lack of natural rewards. Understanding this syndrome provides insights into the diverse pathways that lead to addiction.

The Pre-frontal Cortex: Executive Control Impaired

The pre-frontal cortex, responsible for executive functions such as decision-making and impulse control, plays a critical role in addiction. This chapter explores how substance use impairs the pre-frontal cortex, diminishing an individual's ability to make reasoned decisions and resist impulses. The compromised executive control further entrenches the cycle of addiction.

Hijacking the Brain's Survival Mechanisms: The Vicious Cycle

Substances, through their impact on the brain's reward system, effectively hijack the same mechanisms designed to ensure survival. Chapter 4 examines how addiction tricks the brain into prioritizing substances over essential needs, perpetuating a vicious cycle where the pursuit of pleasure takes precedence over fundamental aspects of well-being.

Dual Diagnosis: Mental Health and Addiction

The interplay between mental health and addiction is a complex facet of the neurobiology of substance dependence. This chapter explores the bidirectional relationship, elucidating how mental health disorders can contribute to the vulnerability to addiction and, conversely, how substance use can exacerbate existing mental health challenges. Recognizing this dual diagnosis is essential for comprehensive treatment approaches.

Withdrawal and Cravings: The Battle Within

The neurobiology of addiction comes to the forefront during withdrawal, a challenging phase where the brain, accustomed to the presence of substances, reacts to their absence. This chapter navigates the physiological processes underlying withdrawal symptoms and cravings. Understanding this battle within the brain is crucial for individuals seeking recovery, as it sheds light on the formidable challenges they may face.

Genetic Predisposition: Unrevealing the Code

Genetic factors contribute significantly to an individual's susceptibility to addiction. Chapter 4 delves into the intricate genetic landscape, exploring how specific genes may predispose some individuals to substance dependence. Recognizing genetic predisposition underscores the importance of personalized approaches to addiction treatment.

From Tolerance to Dependence: Gradual Escalation

The neurobiology of addiction provides insights into the gradual escalation from tolerance to dependence. This chapter traces the trajectory, explaining how repeated exposure to substances prompts the brain to adapt, leading to increased tolerance and, ultimately, dependence. Understanding this progression is key to dismantling the illusion of control that often accompanies early substance use.

Conclusion of Chapter 4:

As readers conclude their exploration of "The Neurobiology of Addiction," they emerge with a profound understanding of the intricate mechanisms that underlie substance dependence. This chapter is not merely a scientific inquiry; it is an illumination—a spotlight on the biological forces that shape the journey into addiction. Armed with this knowledge, individuals are empowered to approach recovery with a deeper understanding of the neurobiological challenges they face, fostering a sense of agency in the pursuit of breaking free from the chains of addiction.

Chapter 5: Societal Impact and Stigma

In the complex tapestry of addiction, societal perceptions and stigma cast profound shadows, influencing the experiences of individuals grappling with substance dependence. Chapter 5, "Societal Impact and Stigma," embarks on an exploration of the external forces that shape the narrative of addiction, shedding light on the impact of societal norms, judgement, and the pervasive stigma that veils this often-misunderstood struggle.

The Weight of Societal Norms: Unseen Influences

Societal norms act as silent architects, shaping the lens through which addiction is perceived. This chapter delves into the subtle influences of cultural expectations and prevailing attitudes toward substance use. By unrevealing these unseen forces, readers gain insights into the societal backdrop that can either foster understanding or contribute to the perpetuation of stigma.

Judgement and Morality: The Interplay with Addiction

Moral judgement often become entwined with discussions of addiction, introducing an additional layer of complexity. Chapter 5 navigates the interplay between societal perceptions of morality and addiction, exploring how moralistic viewpoints can impact individuals, hindering open conversations and perpetuating the cycle of shame.

Language Matters: The Power of Discourse

The words we choose to describe addiction wield significant influence. This chapter underscores the power of language in shaping societal attitudes and examines the impact of stigmatizing terminology. By recognizing the role of discourse, readers are encouraged to engage in conversations that foster empathy and destigmatize the language surrounding addiction.

The Hidden Faces of Addiction: Demographics and Bias

Societal impact is not uniform, and biases can manifest in varied ways. This chapter explores how demographic factors, including race, gender, and socio-economic status, intersect with addiction, influencing the experiences of individuals. By acknowledging these hidden faces of addiction, readers gain a broader understanding of the diverse narratives within this complex landscape.

The Ripple Effect: Families and Communities

Addiction reverberates beyond the individual, affecting families and communities. Chapter 5 examines the societal impact through the lens of familial and communal dynamics. The stigma surrounding addiction can isolate individuals and hinder support systems, contributing to a cycle of secrecy that exacerbates the challenges of recovery.

Media Portrayals: Shaping Perceptions

Media plays a pivotal role in shaping public perceptions of addiction. This chapter scrutinizes how media portrayals contribute to societal attitudes and stigma surrounding substance dependence. By dissecting the narratives presented in various forms of media, readers gain awareness of the potential impact on public understanding and empathy.

Legislation and Policies: Navigating the Legal Landscape

Societal impact extends to legislative and policy realms, influencing the availability of resources for addiction treatment and shaping legal approaches. This chapter navigates the complexities of legislation and policies surrounding addiction, exploring how legal frameworks either support or impede efforts to address the root causes of substance dependence.

Breaking the Silence: Advocacy and Education

While societal impact often perpetuates stigma, advocacy and education serve as powerful tools for change. This chapter illuminates the role of breaking the silence—of individuals and organizations advocating for increased awareness, understanding, and resources. By highlighting initiatives that challenge societal norms, readers are inspired to contribute to the transformative process of dismantling stigma.

Building Empathy: The Antidote to Stigma

Empathy emerges as a potent antidote to stigma. Chapter 5 explores the ways in which building empathy at the individual and societal levels can reshape the narrative of addiction. By fostering understanding and compassion, readers are invited to contribute to a more supportive environment that empowers individuals on their journey to recovery.

Conclusion of Chapter 5:

As readers conclude their exploration of "Societal Impact and Stigma," they are left with a profound awareness of the external forces that shape the experiences of those touched by addiction. This chapter is not merely an analysis of societal dynamics; it is a call to action—a call to challenge stigmatizing norms and foster a climate of empathy and understanding. Armed with this knowledge, readers are empowered to contribute to the transformative process of unmasking addiction, dismantling societal stigma, and supporting individuals on their quest to break free from the chains that bind.

Chapter 6: Recognizing Early Signs

In the labyrinth of addiction, early recognition becomes a beacon of hope—a crucial tool in the journey towards recovery. Chapter 6, "Recognizing Early Signs," unveils the subtle indicators that may signal the onset of addictive behaviours. By navigating the landscape of early signs, readers are equipped with the knowledge to intervene, fostering a greater likelihood of successful recovery.

Subtle Shifts in Behaviour: The Prelude to Awareness

The chapter begins by illuminating the subtle shifts in behaviour that often precede full-fledged addiction. From alterations in social patterns to changes in priorities, these early signs serve as whispers—a prelude to a deeper awareness. By acknowledging and understanding these shifts, individuals and their support networks gain a valuable window into the unfolding narrative of addiction.

Fluctuations in Mood and Energy: A Tell-tale Terrain

Early signs of addiction often manifest in fluctuations in mood and energy levels. This chapter delves into the intricacies of these tell-tale indicators, exploring how shifts from euphoria to lethargy or irritability can be early glimpses into the impact of substances on an individual's emotional well-being. Recognizing these fluctuations becomes instrumental in deciphering the language of early signs.

Social Isolation and Withdrawal: Red Flags Unveiled

Isolation and withdrawal from social connections are common companions of addiction's early stages. Chapter 6 unravels the significance of these red flags, examining how individuals may gradually distance themselves from friends, family, or activities they once enjoyed. By recognizing the social dimensions of early signs, readers are empowered to initiate conversations and offer support.

Changes in Priorities: Unravelling Shifts in Focus

The recalibration of priorities is another pivotal early sign that warrants attention. This chapter scrutinizes how individuals may undergo subtle shifts in focus, with substances gradually taking precedence over personal, professional, or relational obligations. Understanding these changes in priorities provides insight into the evolving dynamics of addiction's early stages.

Performance and Academic Decline: Navigating the Impact

For those in academic or professional settings, early signs of addiction may manifest in a decline in performance. This chapter explores how individuals may struggle to maintain previous levels of achievement, with addiction exerting its influence on concentration, motivation, and overall functioning. Recognizing these academic and performance-related shifts is crucial for timely intervention.

Financial Strain: Tracing the Ripples

The ripples of addiction often extend to financial realms. Chapter 6 examines how individuals grappling with early signs of addiction may experience financial strain due to increased spending on substances or a decline in productivity affecting income. By tracing these financial ripples, readers gain a holistic understanding of the impact of addiction on various facets of life.

Changes in Physical Appearance: The Mirror of Warning

The mirror becomes a metaphor for early signs of addiction as changes in physical appearance may serve as visible warnings. This chapter explores how factors like weight loss, changes in grooming habits, or the emergence of health issues can be indicative of underlying substance use. Recognizing these physical transformations becomes a tangible step in acknowledging early signs.

Defensive Behaviour: Shields Against Scrutiny

Individuals in the early stages of addiction often erect defensive shields to protect their evolving behaviour. Chapter 6 dissects these defensive mechanisms, exploring how individuals may deflect questions, minimize concerns, or become secretive about their activities. Understanding this defensive behaviour is instrumental in approaching conversations with sensitivity and empathy.

Inconsistencies in Communication: Cracks in the Facade

Communication inconsistencies emerge as cracks in the facade of early-stage addiction. This chapter navigates how individuals may struggle to maintain coherent or honest communication, resorting to deception or avoidance. Recognizing these subtle communication shifts allows readers to pierce through the veil of addiction and establish connections based on transparency and trust.

Conclusion of Chapter 6:

As readers conclude their exploration of "Recognizing Early Signs," they emerge with a heightened sensitivity to the nuanced indicators that precede addiction's full manifestation. This chapter is not merely a catalogue of behaviours; it is an invitation to vigilance—a call to recognize the whispers before they become shouts. Armed with the insights gained, readers are empowered to navigate the delicate terrain of early signs, fostering an environment where intervention becomes a bridge to recovery, and the chains of addiction can be loosened before they tighten their grip.

Chapter 7: Personal Stories of Unmasking

In the symphony of addiction, personal narratives resonate as powerful chords that weave through the fabric of shared experience. Chapter 7, "Personal Stories of Unmasking," takes a deeply personal turn as real-life accounts unfold. These narratives serve as beacons of hope, shedding light on the transformative journey from the clutches of addiction to the courageous unveiling of one's true self.

Voices of Resilience: Breaking the Silence

The chapter begins by amplifying the voices of resilience—individuals who, through vulnerability and courage, have chosen to break the silence surrounding their struggles with addiction. These stories transcend statistics and stereotypes, offering readers an intimate glimpse into the complexities, challenges, and triumphs that mark the path of unmasking addiction.

From Darkness to Light: Navigating the Shadows

Personal stories often navigate the shadows, traversing the tumultuous journey from darkness to light. Chapter 7 delves into narratives that explore the initial encounters with substances, the allure that masked underlying pain, and the gradual realization that unmasking addiction required confronting the shadows within. These stories unveil the raw, unfiltered realities of the battle against addiction.

The Impact on Relationships: Shattered and Rebuilt

Intertwined with personal narratives are the intricate threads of relationships. The chapter examines stories where addiction cast shadows on connections with loved ones—straining bonds, shattering trust, and creating emotional turbulence. Yet, amidst the wreckage, these stories reveal the resilient spirit that seeks to rebuild and repair, demonstrating the transformative power of recovery on interpersonal connections.

Turning Points: Catalysts for Change

Within personal narratives, turning points emerge as catalysts for change. This chapter explores stories where individuals reached pivotal moments—moments that spurred self-reflection, a recognition of the need for change, and the courage to embark on the journey of unmasking addiction. These turning points become beacons that guide others towards their own potential for transformation.

The Role of Support Systems: Anchors in the Storm

Support systems play a pivotal role in the unmasking process. Chapter 7 unfolds stories of individuals who found anchors in the storm—whether through family, friends, or professional networks. These narratives illustrate the profound impact of supportive relationships in fostering resilience and providing the scaffolding for recovery.

Resilience in Relapse: Navigating Setbacks

Not all paths to recovery are linear. The chapter acknowledges the resilience within stories that include relapse—an often-challenging aspect of the unmasking journey. These narratives illuminate the nuanced nature of recovery, demonstrating how setbacks can be transformed into opportunities for growth and renewed commitment to the path of unmasking addiction.

Personal Transformations: Embracing Authenticity

At the core of personal stories of unmasking lies the theme of transformation. This chapter explores narratives of individuals who, through recovery, embraced authenticity—shedding the layers of addiction to reveal their true selves. These stories inspire and illustrate the profound metamorphosis that occurs when individuals courageously unmask the elements that once concealed their authentic identity.

The Journey to Recovery: A Continuing Narrative

While personal stories serve as poignant snapshots, they are also part of a continuing narrative. The chapter emphasizes that the journey to recovery is an ongoing process, marked by growth, self-discovery, and the perpetual commitment to unmasking addiction. These narratives offer a glimpse into the evolving nature of recovery and the resilience required to navigate its twists and turns.

The Power of Shared Experience: Fostering Connection

Personal stories of unmasking addiction underscore the power of shared experience. This chapter explores how these narratives foster connection—bridging the gap between those who have walked the path of recovery and those who may be just beginning. Through shared experiences, a sense of community and understanding blossoms, offering solace and encouragement to those still grappling with the chains of addiction.

Conclusion of Chapter 7:

As readers conclude their immersion in "Personal Stories of Unmasking," they carry with them the echoes of resilience, transformation, and shared humanity. This chapter is not merely a collection of narratives; it is a mosaic—a testament to the diversity of experiences within the realm of addiction and recovery. Armed with the insights gained from these personal stories, readers are invited to reflect on their own journeys, fostering empathy, understanding, and a collective commitment to unmasking addiction's grip on individuals and communities alike.

Book 2: "The Science Behind Addiction: Demystifying the Grip"

Chapter 8: Brain Chemistry and Addiction

In the intricate dance between mind and substance, the landscape of addiction is etched into the very fabric of brain chemistry. Chapter 8, "Brain Chemistry and Addiction," unveils the complex interplay of neurotransmitters, receptors, and neural circuits that underlie the grip of addiction. By dissecting the science behind addiction, readers embark on a journey to demystify the intricacies of the brain's response to substances and the profound impact on behaviour.

Neurotransmitters as Messengers: The Language of the Brain

At the core of brain chemistry lies the language of neurotransmitters—chemical messengers that facilitate communication between neurons. This chapter delves into the role of neurotransmitters such as dopamine, serotonin, and norepinephrine in orchestrating essential functions within the brain. Understanding this intricate language sets the stage for unravelling how substances can hijack these pathways, giving rise to the allure of addiction.

Dopamine: The Pleasure Pathway

Dopamine, often referred to as the "pleasure neurotransmitter," takes centre stage in the addiction narrative. Chapter 8 navigates the dopamine pathway, exploring how the brain's reward system responds to pleasurable stimuli. It illuminates the role of dopamine in reinforcing behaviours that promote survival and how substances, by artificially elevating dopamine levels, create a powerful reward signal that becomes entwined with addictive patterns.

Reward Circuitry: The Neural Symphony

The neural symphony of addiction unfolds within the reward circuitry—a complex network of brain regions dedicated to processing pleasurable experiences.

This chapter scrutinizes how substances activate this circuitry, creating an artificial flood of rewards that reinforces the desire for continued substance use. By understanding the neural symphony, readers gain insights into why addiction becomes a compelling and challenging cycle to break.

Neuroadaptation: The Brain's Dance with Change

The brain is a dynamic organ, constantly adapting to its environment. Chapter 8 explores the concept of neuroadaptation, where repeated exposure to substances induces changes in the brain's structure and function. These adaptations contribute to the development of tolerance, where increasing amounts of substances are needed to achieve the same effect, and form the basis of dependence—a hallmark of addiction.

Receptors and Lock-and-Key Mechanisms: Substance Affinities

Substances and the brain engage in a lock-and-key dance mediated by receptors—specialized proteins that bind with neurotransmitters. This chapter unveils the lock-and-key mechanisms, explaining how substances mimic or enhance the actions of natural neurotransmitters. Understanding these affinities provides insight into why certain substances have a profound impact on the brain's chemistry and contribute to addictive behaviours.

Serotonin and Mood Regulation: The Emotional Landscape

Beyond dopamine, serotonin emerges as a key player in the emotional landscape of addiction. Chapter 8 explores how alterations in serotonin levels influence mood regulation and contribute to the development of mental health challenges often co-occurring with addiction. By examining the role of serotonin, readers gain a comprehensive understanding of the intricate connections between brain chemistry, emotions, and addictive behaviours.

GABA and Inhibitory Control: The Brakes on Excitement*

In the orchestration of brain chemistry, gamma-aminobutyric acid (GABA) serves as a crucial conductor, exerting inhibitory control to balance excitatory signals. This chapter dissects the role of GABA in addiction, elucidating how substances can disrupt this balance, leading to heightened excitability and reinforcing addictive patterns. Understanding GABA's role provides a nuanced perspective on the dysregulation inherent in addiction.

Glutamate and Learning: The Path to Cravings

Learning and memory processes within the brain involve the neurotransmitter glutamate. Chapter 8 unravels how glutamate contributes to the formation of cravings—a persistent desire for substances driven by the brain's adaptation to the pleasurable effects of addiction. By exploring glutamate's role, readers gain insights into the mechanisms that perpetuate the cycle of substance use.

The Prefrontal Cortex: Executive Dysfunction in Addiction

The prefrontal cortex, the brain's executive control centre, plays a pivotal role in decision-making and impulse control. This chapter examines how addiction can lead to executive dysfunction, impairing the prefrontal cortex's ability to regulate behaviour and resist impulses. Understanding the impact on executive control provides a lens through which to comprehend the challenges individuals face in breaking free from addictive patterns.

The Role of Genetics: Unravelling the Code

Genetics intersects with brain chemistry, contributing to an individual's susceptibility to addiction. This chapter navigates the intricate genetic landscape, exploring how specific genes may influence the response to substances and the risk of developing addictive behaviours. Recognizing genetic factors underscores the personalized nature of addiction vulnerability.

Neuroplasticity: The Ever-Changing Brain

The brain's ability to adapt, known as neuroplasticity, is a central theme in addiction. Chapter 8 elucidates how repeated exposure to substances induces neuroplastic changes, altering the brain's structure and function. These enduring changes not only reinforce addictive behaviours but also present challenges in the journey to recovery, highlighting the importance of understanding the ever-changing nature of the addicted brain.

Conclusion of Chapter 8:

As readers conclude their exploration of "Brain Chemistry and Addiction," they emerge with a profound understanding of the symphony playing within the neural realms of substance dependence. This chapter is not merely a scientific inquiry; it is an illumination—a spotlight on the intricate dance of neurotransmitters, receptors, and neural pathways that shape the grip of addiction. Armed with this knowledge, readers are empowered to approach addiction with a deeper understanding of the brain's role, fostering a sense of empathy, agency, and a collective commitment to demystifying the complexities that underlie the chains of addiction.

Chapter 9: Genetic Predisposition

In the exploration of addiction's intricate tapestry, the role of genetics emerges as a significant thread, weaving through the fabric of susceptibility and resilience. Chapter 9, "Genetic Predisposition," delves into the complex interplay between genes and addiction, unravelling the genetic landscape that contributes to an individual's vulnerability or resistance to the grip of substances.

The Genetic Blueprint: Unravelling Susceptibility

At the core of genetic predisposition lies the intricate genetic blueprint that each individual inherits. This chapter embarks on the journey of unravelling susceptibility by examining how specific genes influence an individual's response to substances. Understanding the genetic landscape becomes a crucial step in comprehending why some individuals may be more prone to developing addictive behaviours than others.

Heritability of Addiction: Nature vs. Nurture

The interplay between nature and nurture—genetics and environment—forms the backdrop of the heritability of addiction. Chapter 9 navigates the complex dance between genetic predisposition and environmental factors, shedding light on how both contribute to the development of addictive behaviours. Recognizing the nuanced interaction between nature and nurture is essential for a comprehensive understanding of genetic influences on addiction.

Twin, Family, and Adoption Studies: Unmasking Patterns

Twin, family, and adoption studies serve as investigative tools in unmasking the patterns of genetic predisposition. This chapter explores the findings of such studies, revealing the higher likelihood of addiction among individuals with a family history of substance dependence. By examining the evidence from various study designs, readers gain insight into the degree to which genetic factors contribute to addiction risk.

Specific Genes and Risk Alleles: Navigating the Code

Within the vast landscape of genetics, specific genes and risk alleles emerge as focal points of exploration. This chapter delves into the identification of genes associated with addiction vulnerability, such as those involved in neurotransmitter regulation, reward pathways, and impulse control. Navigating the genetic code provides a deeper understanding of the molecular mechanisms that underlie the predisposition to addiction.

Dopamine Receptor Genes: The Pleasure Connection

Dopamine receptor genes take centre stage in the genetic theatre of addiction. Chapter 9 scrutinizes how variations in genes encoding dopamine receptors can influence an individual's responsiveness to pleasurable stimuli, impacting the propensity for addictive behaviours. Understanding the pleasure connection at the genetic level sheds light on why certain individuals may be more drawn to substances that activate the brain's reward system.

Serotonin Transporter Gene: Emotional Resilience

The serotonin transporter gene is another key player in the genetic predisposition to addiction. This chapter explores how variations in this gene can influence serotonin levels, impacting mood regulation and emotional resilience. Recognizing the role of the serotonin transporter gene provides insights into the complex interactions between genetic factors, emotional well-being, and the development of addictive behaviours.

GABA Receptor Genes: Inhibitory Control Unveiled

In the intricate dance of genetic predisposition, GABA receptor genes reveal the story of inhibitory control.

Chapter 9 dissects how variations in genes related to gamma-aminobutyric acid (GABA) receptors can impact the brain's ability to exert inhibitory control, contributing to heightened excitability and susceptibility to addictive patterns. Understanding GABA receptor genes adds a layer of complexity to the genetic landscape of addiction.

Opioid Receptor Genes: Unravelling the Opium of Addiction

Opioid receptor genes, central to the brain's response to endorphins and exogenous opioids, play a crucial role in addiction vulnerability. This chapter navigates the genetic variations in opioid receptor genes, explaining how these variations can influence an individual's sensitivity to the rewarding effects of opioids. Unravelling the opium of addiction at the genetic level provides a deeper understanding of the pathways that contribute to opioid dependence.

Alcohol Metabolism Genes: Enzymatic Influences

Genetic predisposition to alcohol dependence involves the interplay of alcohol metabolism genes. This chapter examines how variations in genes responsible for alcohol metabolism can impact an individual's sensitivity to alcohol, influencing the risk of developing alcohol use disorders. Recognizing the enzymatic influences on alcohol metabolism adds a biochemical layer to the genetic factors associated with alcohol addiction.

Complex Interactions: Polygenic Nature of Addiction

The polygenic nature of addiction emphasizes that multiple genes, each contributing a modest effect, collectively influence susceptibility. This chapter explores the complexity of interactions between various genes associated with addiction, illustrating how the cumulative impact of multiple genetic factors shapes an individual's predisposition. Recognizing the polygenic nature underscores the multifaceted genetic landscape of addiction.

Epigenetics: The Symphony of Gene Expression

Beyond the genetic code lies the symphony of epigenetics—the dynamic modulation of gene expression influenced by environmental factors. Chapter 9 delves into the epigenetic mechanisms that modify the activity of genes related to addiction susceptibility. Understanding how environmental factors can shape gene expression adds a layer of adaptability to the genetic predisposition narrative.

Personalized Approaches to Treatment: Tailoring Interventions

The recognition of genetic predisposition paves the way for personalized approaches to addiction treatment. This chapter explores how understanding an individual's genetic profile can inform tailored interventions, optimizing the efficacy of treatment strategies. Recognizing the unique genetic makeup of each individual opens avenues for precision medicine in the field of addiction.

Conclusion of Chapter 9:

As readers conclude their exploration of "Genetic Predisposition," they emerge with a nuanced understanding of the intricate genetic landscape that shapes vulnerability to addiction. This chapter is not merely a catalogue of genes; it is an exploration—an illumination into the molecular symphony that underlies the predisposition to addictive behaviours. Armed with this knowledge, readers are empowered to comprehend the diversity of genetic influences, fostering a sense of empathy, and contributing to a more comprehensive understanding of addiction's grip on individuals and the potential for tailored interventions in the pursuit of breaking free from its chains.

Chapter 10: Environmental Factors

In the intricate interplay between genes and the environment, Chapter 10, "Environmental Factors," unfolds as a pivotal exploration into the external influences that shape the trajectory of addiction. This chapter delves into the multifaceted role of the environment—ranging from early life experiences to societal influences—in contributing to the development of addictive behaviours and influencing the complex dance of susceptibility and resilience.

Early Life Experiences: The Foundation of Vulnerability
The journey into environmental factors commences with the foundational impact of early life experiences. This chapter scrutinizes how factors such as childhood trauma, adverse events, and the quality of caregiving can imprint lasting impressions on an individual's vulnerability to addiction. Understanding the roots of susceptibility in early experiences sets the stage for unravelling the intricate dynamics between environmental factors and addiction.

Family Dynamics: The Crucible of Influence

Within the realm of environmental factors, family dynamics emerge as a crucible of influence. Chapter 10 navigates the intricate relationships and communication patterns within families that contribute to the development of addictive behaviours. It explores how familial factors, including parenting styles, family history of addiction, and the presence of substance use within the family, shape an individual's perception of substances and influence their risk of addiction.

Peer Influence: Navigating Social Currents

The social currents of peer influence become a focal point in understanding environmental factors. This chapter delves into how interactions with peers, social norms, and the desire for social acceptance can impact an individual's engagement with substances. By navigating the influence of peer relationships, readers gain insights into the external forces that shape the choices individuals make in the context of addiction.

School and Academic Environment: Stressors and Coping Mechanisms

The academic environment unfolds as a backdrop where stressors and coping mechanisms intersect. Chapter 10 explores how academic stress, peer relationships within school settings, and the availability of substances in educational environments can influence vulnerability to addiction. Understanding the role of the academic milieu provides a comprehensive perspective on the environmental factors that contribute to the complex tapestry of addiction.

Socio-economic Status: Disparities and Challenges

Environmental factors extend to socioeconomic status, unveiling disparities and challenges that impact addiction risk. This chapter navigates how economic factors, access to resources, and disparities in opportunities can shape an individual's susceptibility to addictive behaviours. Recognizing the role of socioeconomic status provides a lens through which to comprehend the broader societal influences that contribute to the grip of addiction.

Cultural and Societal Norms: The Canvas of Influence

The canvas of cultural and societal norms becomes a backdrop against which environmental influences unfold. Chapter 10 scrutinizes how cultural attitudes toward substance use, societal expectations, and prevailing norms can shape an individual's perception of substances and influence the risk of addiction. By navigating these cultural currents, readers gain insights into the external forces that mold the landscape of addiction vulnerability.

Media and Advertising: Shaping Perceptions

In the digital age, media and advertising wield considerable influence over perceptions of substances. This chapter explores how media portrayals, advertising strategies, and the accessibility of substance-related content impact individuals, particularly the younger demographic. Understanding the role of media in shaping perceptions sheds light on the environmental factors that contribute to the allure of substances.

Access to Substances: The Physical Landscape

The physical landscape of access to substances emerges as a tangible environmental factor. Chapter 10 delves into how the availability of substances in communities, neighbourhoods, and social circles can influence an individual's likelihood of engaging in substance use. Recognizing the impact of physical access provides insights into the external elements that contribute to the development of addictive behaviours.

Stress and Coping Mechanisms: Adaptive Responses

Stress, a ubiquitous aspect of the human experience, becomes a key player in the environmental factors that influence addiction. This chapter explores how exposure to chronic stressors, adverse life events, and the lack of healthy coping mechanisms can shape an individual's vulnerability to addiction. Understanding stress as an environmental factor sheds light on adaptive responses that may lead to the reliance on substances as coping mechanisms.

Trauma and Post-Traumatic Stress: The Lingering Shadows

Environmental factors extend to the shadows of trauma and post-traumatic stress. Chapter 10 examines how experiences of trauma, whether physical, emotional, or psychological, can contribute to the development of addictive behaviours as individuals seek relief from lingering distress. Recognizing trauma as an environmental factor provides a deeper understanding of the complexities that underlie addiction.

Community and Social Support: Protective Factors

Amidst the myriad influences, community and social support emerge as protective factors within the environmental landscape. This chapter explores how a strong sense of community, positive social relationships, and access to support networks can mitigate the impact of other environmental stressors, serving as buffers against addiction. Recognizing the role of social support underscores the potential for resilience in the face of challenging environmental factors.

Prevention and Intervention Strategies: Navigating Environmental Influences

The recognition of environmental factors opens avenues for prevention and intervention strategies. This chapter explores how understanding and addressing environmental influences can inform targeted interventions. By navigating the environmental landscape, readers gain insights into the potential for mitigating addiction risk through community-based initiatives, educational programs, and the cultivation of supportive environments.

****Conclusion of Chapter 10: ****

As readers conclude their exploration of "Environmental Factors," they emerge with a comprehensive understanding of the external influences that mold the landscape of addiction vulnerability. This chapter is not merely an analysis of environmental elements; it is an invitation—an invitation to recognize the intricate dance between the individual and their surroundings. Armed with this knowledge, readers are empowered to navigate the environmental factors that contribute to the grip of addiction, fostering a sense of agency, and contributing to a more comprehensive understanding of the external forces at play in the complex tapestry of addictive behaviours.

Chapter 11: Dual Diagnosis: Mental Health and Addiction

In the intricate web of addiction, Chapter 11, "Dual Diagnosis: Mental Health and Addiction," unfolds as a poignant exploration into the convergence of mental health and substance use disorders. This chapter delves into the complex interplay between psychological well-being and addictive behaviours, unravelling the challenges, nuances, and treatment considerations that arise when mental health and addiction coexist within the same individual.

The Coexistence of Mental Health and Addiction: A Complex Nexus

At the heart of dual diagnosis lies the complex nexus where mental health and addiction converge. This chapter begins by elucidating the coexistence of mental health disorders, such as depression, anxiety, bipolar disorder, or post-traumatic stress disorder (PTSD), with substance use disorders. Understanding the interplay between these two realms lays the foundation for navigating the intricate challenges inherent in dual diagnosis.

Common Comorbidities: Mapping the Landscape

Dual diagnosis is marked by a landscape of common comorbidities—instances where mental health disorders and substance use disorders intersect. Chapter 11 maps this landscape, exploring the prevalence of specific mental health conditions alongside different types of substance misuse. By examining the patterns of comorbidity, readers gain insights into the multifaceted nature of dual diagnosis and the diverse ways in which mental health and addiction intertwine.

Bidirectional Influence: The Reciprocal Relationship

The relationship between mental health and addiction is bidirectional, with each influencing the course of the other. This chapter scrutinizes how mental health challenges may contribute to the development or exacerbation of substance use disorders, while substance use, in turn, can impact mental health outcomes. Understanding the reciprocal nature of this relationship provides a nuanced perspective on the dynamics within dual diagnosis.

Self-Medication and Coping Strategies: Unveiling Motivations

Individuals experiencing mental health challenges within the realm of dual diagnosis often resort to self-medication as a coping strategy. Chapter 11 unveils the motivations behind self-medication, exploring how substances may be used to alleviate symptoms, numb emotional pain, or provide a temporary escape. Recognizing these motivations sheds light on the underlying needs that drive individuals toward the complex terrain of dual diagnosis.

Increased Vulnerability: Shared Risk Factors

Dual diagnosis is characterized by shared risk factors that increase an individual's vulnerability to both mental health and substance use disorders. This chapter navigates these shared risk factors, including genetic predisposition, early life adversity, trauma, and environmental stressors. By recognizing the overlapping vulnerabilities, readers gain a holistic understanding of the factors that contribute to the intertwined nature of mental health and addiction.

Neurobiological Interactions: The Impact on Brain Chemistry

The neurobiological interactions within dual diagnosis unfold as a key aspect of the chapter.

It explores how substances and mental health disorders can both impact brain chemistry, leading to complex alterations in neurotransmitter systems and neural circuits. Understanding the neurobiological

Underpinnings provides insight into the intricacies of dual diagnosis and the challenges posed by the simultaneous involvement of mental health and addiction in the brain's landscape.

Diagnostic Challenges: Navigating Complexity

Diagnosing and assessing dual diagnosis poses unique challenges due to the complexity of symptoms and overlapping manifestations. Chapter 11 delves into the diagnostic challenges that clinicians face when mental health and substance use disorders coexist. It explores the nuances of symptom presentation, the potential for masking or exacerbating conditions, and the importance of comprehensive assessments to unravel the complexity within dual diagnosis.

Integrated Treatment Approaches: A Holistic Framework

Treatment approaches for dual diagnosis embrace an integrated, holistic framework that addresses both mental health and addiction simultaneously. This chapter navigates the landscape of integrated treatment, exploring therapeutic modalities that consider the interconnected nature of these disorders. From psychotherapy and medication management to support groups and lifestyle interventions, integrated approaches provide a comprehensive tool-kit for addressing the diverse needs of individuals with dual diagnosis.

Recovery Challenges: Breaking the Cycle

Individuals grappling with dual diagnosis often face unique challenges on the path to recovery. Chapter 11 examines these challenges, including the potential for relapse, difficulties in medication adherence, and the need for ongoing mental health support. By understanding the specific hurdles within dual diagnosis recovery, readers gain insights into the complexities that individuals must navigate in breaking free from the cycle of mental health challenges and substance use.

Relapse Prevention: Targeting Triggers and Vulnerabilities

Relapse prevention within dual diagnosis involves targeting triggers and vulnerabilities specific to both mental health and addiction. This chapter explores strategies for identifying and addressing these triggers, encompassing elements such as stress management, coping skills development, and the creation of a robust support network. Recognizing the intricacies of relapse prevention contributes to a more nuanced approach in supporting individuals with dual diagnosis.

Community and Peer Support: A Vital Network

Communuity and peer support play a vital role in the journey of individuals with dual diagnosis. Chapter 11 examines the significance of these networks, including mutual aid groups, peer-led initiatives, and community-based resources. By recognizing the importance of community and peer support, readers gain an appreciation for the collaborative efforts needed to foster resilience and sustained recovery within the realm of dual diagnosis.

Conclusion of Chapter 11:

As readers conclude their exploration of "Dual Diagnosis: Mental Health and Addiction," they emerge with a profound understanding of the intricate interplay between psychological well-being and substance use disorders. This chapter is not merely an analysis of coexisting conditions; it is an acknowledgement—an acknowledgement of the complex challenges faced by individuals navigating the terrain of dual diagnosis. Armed with insights into the bidirectional influences, shared risk factors, and the reciprocal relationship between mental health and addiction, readers are empowered to approach dual diagnosis with compassion, empathy, and a holistic perspective. The journey through this chapter not only sheds light on the complexities of dual diagnosis but also underscores the importance of integrated treatment approaches, personalized interventions, and the supportive networks that contribute to breaking free from the entwining grip of mental health challenges and substance use disorders. In recognizing the resilience within those facing dual diagnosis, this chapter serves as a call to action—a call to foster understanding, destigmatize these intertwined struggles, and contribute to a more compassionate and effective approach to supporting individuals on their journey to recovery.

Chapter 12: Impact on Cognitive Function

In the intricate tapestry of addiction, Chapter 12, "Impact on Cognitive Function," unfolds as a crucial exploration into the profound effects that substance use can exert on the cognitive abilities of individuals. This chapter delves into the intricate interplay between addiction and cognitive function, unveiling how substances can alter the neural landscape, impair decision-making, and compromise various facets of cognitive processing.

Neurological Impact: Rewiring the Brain's Circuitry*

The journey into the impact on cognitive function begins with an examination of the neurological changes induced by substances. Chapter 12 scrutinizes how repeated exposure to drugs or alcohol can lead to neuroadaptations, altering the connectivity and function of neural circuits involved in cognition. Understanding the neurological impact provides insights into the mechanisms through which substances can reshape the brain's circuitry, setting the stage for cognitive consequences.

Executive Functions: The Frontal Lobe's Role

Executive functions, governed by the frontal lobe of the brain, play a pivotal role in cognitive control and decision-making. This chapter navigates how addiction can compromise executive functions, impairing abilities such as impulse control, planning, and judgement. By exploring the frontal lobe's role in executive functions, readers gain a nuanced understanding of how substance use can disrupt the cognitive processes essential for adaptive and goal-directed behaviour.

Memory Impairment: The Fragility of Recall

Memory, a cornerstone of cognitive function, becomes susceptible to the impact of substance use. Chapter 12 examines how addiction can lead to memory impairment, affecting both short-term and long-term memory systems. It unveils the fragility of recall as substances interfere with the encoding, consolidation, and retrieval of information, contributing to cognitive challenges among individuals grappling with addiction.

Attention and Concentration: The Flickering Focus

Attention and concentration, essential components of cognitive function, face disruption within the realm of addiction. This chapter delves into how substances can lead to a flickering focus, impairing sustained attention and the ability to concentrate on tasks. By exploring the impact on attentional processes, readers gain insights into the cognitive challenges that individuals with addiction may encounter in their daily lives.

Processing Speed: The Sluggish Stride

Processing speed, reflecting the efficiency of cognitive operations, can experience a sluggish stride in the presence of substance use. Chapter 12 navigates how addiction can compromise the speed at which individuals process information, impacting reaction times and cognitive efficiency. Understanding the consequences for processing speed sheds light on the multifaceted nature of cognitive impairment within the context of addiction.

Decision-Making and Impulsivity: A Delicate Balance

The delicate balance between decision-making and impulsivity becomes disrupted in the wake of addiction. This chapter scrutinizes how substances can tilt this balance, leading to impulsive behaviours and compromised decision-making processes. By exploring the intricate interplay between addiction and impulsivity, readers gain insights into the challenges individuals face in making adaptive choices that align with long-term goals.

Emotional Regulation: Turmoil and Dysregulation

Emotional regulation, intertwined with cognitive function, faces turmoil and dysregulation in the presence of substance use. Chapter 12 delves into how addiction can impact the ability to regulate emotions effectively, contributing to mood swings, heightened reactivity, and difficulties in coping with stress. Recognizing the emotional dimensions of cognitive impairment adds a layer of complexity to understanding the holistic impact of addiction on cognitive function.

Neurocognitive Testing: Unveiling Deficits

The assessment of cognitive function through neurocognitive testing serves as a valuable tool in unveiling deficits associated with addiction. This chapter explores the methodologies and findings of such testing, shedding light on specific cognitive domains affected by substance use. By examining neurocognitive deficits, readers gain a quantitative understanding of the cognitive challenges individuals may experience as a result of addiction.

Long-Term Consequences: The Lingering Shadows

The impact of substance use on cognitive function extends beyond immediate effects, casting lingering shadows over the long term. This chapter navigates the long-term consequences of addiction, exploring how persistent substance use can lead to enduring cognitive deficits. Recognizing the enduring nature of these consequences underscores the importance of early intervention and comprehensive approaches to mitigating cognitive impairment.

Cognitive Reserve: Understanding Variability

Cognitive reserve, reflecting an individual's ability to withstand and recover from cognitive challenges, becomes a focal point in understanding variability within the impact of addiction on cognitive function. This chapter examines the concept of cognitive reserve, exploring how factors such as education, intellectual engagement, and lifestyle choices may influence the degree to which individuals are resilient in the face of cognitive impairment associated with substance use.

Recovery and Cognitive Rehabilitation: Nurturing Renewal

Recovery from addiction opens avenues for cognitive rehabilitation and nurturing cognitive renewal. This chapter explores strategies and interventions aimed at supporting individuals in reclaiming cognitive function during the recovery journey. From cognitive-behavioural therapies to lifestyle modifications, the chapter highlights the potential for fostering cognitive resilience and promoting cognitive health as part of the recovery process.

Public Health Implications: A Call for Awareness

The impact of addiction on cognitive function holds significant public health implications. Chapter 12 examines the broader consequences for society, including the potential strain on healthcare systems, economic productivity, and the need for awareness and education. Recognizing the public health dimensions of cognitive impairment due to addiction underscores the importance of preventive measures, early intervention, and comprehensive strategies for addressing the cognitive consequences at a societal level.

Conclusion of Chapter 12:

As readers conclude their exploration of "Impact on Cognitive Function," they emerge with a profound understanding of the intricate relationship between substance use and cognitive impairment. This chapter is not merely an analysis of deficits; it is a testament—an acknowledgement of the multifaceted challenges faced by individuals grappling with addiction. Armed with insights into the neurological impact, disruptions to executive functions, and the enduring consequences for cognitive function, readers are empowered to approach addiction with a comprehensive perspective. The journey through this chapter not only sheds light on the complexities of cognitive impairment associated with substance use but also underscores the importance of early intervention, cognitive rehabilitation, and a collective commitment to addressing the impact on cognitive function as part of the broader landscape of addiction. In recognizing the cognitive dimensions of addiction, this chapter serves as a call to action—a call to foster awareness, destigmatize cognitive challenges, and contribute to a more informed and compassionate approach to supporting individuals on their journey to recovery from the intricate web of addiction's impact on cognitive functio

Chapter 13: Neuroplasticity and Recovery

In the intricate dance between addiction and recovery, Chapter 13, "Neuroplasticity and Recovery," unfolds as a beacon of hope and understanding. This chapter delves into the remarkable phenomenon of neuroplasticity—the brain's capacity to adapt and reorganize itself—and its profound implications for individuals on the path to recovery from addiction. It explores how the brain's resilience, coupled with intentional interventions, can pave the way for transformative changes, fostering renewal and rebuilding in the wake of substance use.

Neuroplasticity Unveiled: The Brain's Adaptive Symphony

The exploration of neuroplasticity begins with an unveiling of the brain's adaptive symphony. Chapter 13 scrutinizes the dynamic processes through which the brain reshapes itself in response to experiences, learning, and environmental stimuli. Understanding neuroplasticity provides a foundation for appreciating the potential for change and growth within the neural landscapes altered by addiction.

Rewiring Neural Circuits: A Journey of Transformation

Neuroplasticity manifests as the rewiring of neural circuits—a journey of transformation within the brain's intricate architecture. This chapter navigates how intentional interventions, such as cognitive-behavioural therapies, mindfulness practices, and abstinence, can contribute to rewiring neural pathways affected by substance use. By exploring the mechanisms through which neural circuits adapt, readers gain insights into the malleability of the brain on the road to recovery.

Learning and Unlearning: Breaking Habits

The process of recovery involves both learning and unlearning—breaking free from ingrained habits and acquiring new, healthier patterns of behaviour. Chapter 13 delves into how neuroplasticity facilitates the learning and unlearning processes, allowing individuals to reshape their responses to triggers, cravings, and maladaptive coping mechanisms. Understanding the plasticity of the brain's learning mechanisms sheds light on the potential for lasting change in the journey to recovery.

Environmental Enrichment: Nurturing Growth

Environmental enrichment becomes a key player in leveraging neuroplasticity for recovery. This chapter examines how a supportive and stimulating environment can enhance neuroplastic processes, promoting cognitive, emotional, and social growth. By recognizing the impact of environmental factors on neuroplasticity, readers gain insights into the importance of creating a nurturing context that fosters recovery and renewal.

Mindfulness and Meditation: Cultivating Awareness

Mindfulness and meditation emerge as powerful tools for harnessing neuroplasticity in the recovery process. Chapter 13 navigates how these practices, rooted in focused attention and present-moment awareness, can induce structural and functional changes in the brain. Exploring the neuroplastic effects of mindfulness sheds light on how cultivating awareness can be a transformative force in breaking free from the grip of addiction.

Physical Exercise: Energizing the Brain

The role of physical exercise in energizing the brain and supporting neuroplasticity comes to the forefront. This chapter scrutinizes how aerobic exercise, strength training, and movement can enhance the release of neurotrophic factors, fostering neuronal growth and connectivity. Understanding the neuroplastic benefits of physical activity underscores the holistic approach to recovery that encompasses both mental and physical well-being.

Social Connection: Neural Harmony in Relationships

Social connection, a fundamental aspect of human experience, contributes to neural harmony within the context of recovery. Chapter 13 explores how meaningful relationships, support networks, and positive social interactions can influence neuroplasticity, promoting emotional regulation and resilience. Recognizing the neural underpinnings of social connection highlights the importance of community and relationships in the recovery journey.

Neurofeedback and Brain Training: Precision Interventions

Precision interventions, such as neurofeedback and brain training, leverage neuroplasticity for targeted therapeutic outcomes. This chapter delves into how these techniques, utilizing real-time feedback and cognitive exercises, can modulate neural activity and enhance adaptive changes. By exploring the precision of neurofeedback, readers gain insights into the potential for tailored approaches that align with individual needs in the pursuit of recovery.

Epigenetics and Recovery: Modulating Gene Expression

Beyond neuroplasticity lies the symphony of epigenetics—the modulation of gene expression influenced by experiences and environmental factors. Chapter 13 examines how recovery-focused interventions can impact gene expression, contributing to enduring changes in the brain. Understanding the epigenetic dimensions of recovery underscores the lasting influence of intentional interventions on the molecular landscape of addiction.

Challenges and Resilience: Navigating the Journey

The journey of recovery through neuroplasticity is not without its challenges. This chapter navigates the complexities individuals face, including the potential for setbacks, relapses, and the persistence of cravings. By exploring the challenges within the context of neuroplasticity, readers gain insights into the resilience required to navigate the ebb and flow of the recovery journey.

Personalized Approaches: Tailoring Recovery Strategies

Recognizing the individuality of neural responses, personalized approaches become paramount in tailoring recovery strategies. Chapter 13 explores how understanding an individual's unique neural landscape and adapting interventions accordingly can optimize the effectiveness of recovery strategies. This chapter on

"Neuroplasticity and Recovery" serves as a testament to the transformative potential within the human brain, emphasizing the dynamic and adaptable nature of neural circuits in the face of addiction.

Conclusion of Chapter 13:

As readers conclude their exploration of "Neuroplasticity and Recovery," they emerge with a profound appreciation for the brain's resilience and its capacity for renewal in the journey from addiction to recovery. This chapter is not merely a discussion of neuroscientific concepts; it is an invitation—an invitation to recognize the inherent adaptability of the brain and the transformative potential that lies within intentional interventions. Armed with insights into rewiring neural circuits, the role of mindfulness and environmental enrichment, and the challenges and resilience inherent in the recovery process, readers are empowered to approach addiction recovery with a newfound understanding. The journey through this chapter not only illuminates the scientific underpinnings of neuroplasticity but also underscores the significance of personalized, holistic approaches in supporting individuals on their path to recovery. In recognizing the capacity for change within the neural landscape, this chapter serves as a call to action a call to embrace hope, leverage neuroplasticity as a powerful ally, and contribute to the collective efforts aimed at breaking free from the chains of addiction through the remarkable processes of recovery and neural renewal.

Chapter 14: Breaking the Stigma: Dispelling Myths

In the narrative of addiction, Chapter 14, "Breaking the Stigma: Dispelling Myths," emerges as a crucial exploration into the pervasive misconceptions and societal biases that surround substance use disorders. This chapter aims to dismantle the stigmatization of individuals grappling with addiction, fostering a more compassionate and informed understanding of the complexities inherent in the journey from dependence to recovery.

The Stigma of Addiction: A Barrier to Recovery

The exploration into breaking the stigma begins by recognizing the profound impact it exerts on individuals seeking recovery. Chapter 14 scrutinizes how the stigma of addiction can act as a formidable barrier, hindering individuals from seeking help, disclosing their struggles, and accessing the support necessary for their journey to healing. Understanding the pervasive nature of stigma sets the stage for dispelling myths that contribute to this societal bias.

Myth 1: Addiction is a Choice, not a Disease

One of the prevalent myths surrounding addiction is the misconception that it is a matter of choice rather than a complex disease. This chapter delves into the scientific understanding of addiction as a chronic brain disorder, emphasizing the neurobiological changes that underlie the development and persistence of addictive behaviours. Dispelling the myth of choice fosters empathy and recognition of addiction as a medical condition that warrants comprehensive, evidence-based approaches to treatment and support.

Myth 2: Moral Weakness and Lack of Willpower

The notion of moral weakness and lack of willpower as explanations for addiction perpetuates harmful stereotypes. Chapter 14 navigates through the complexities of willpower within the context of addiction, highlighting the influence of neurobiological factors, genetics, and environmental elements. By dispelling the myth of moral weakness, readers gain insights into the multifaceted nature of addiction and the importance of approaching individuals with empathy and understanding.

Myth 3: Addicts Can't Recover

The perception that individuals grappling with addiction are incapable of recovery perpetuates a sense of hopelessness. This chapter explores the evidence-based reality that recovery from addiction is not only possible but also achievable with the right support and interventions. Dispelling the myth of irreversibility sheds light on the resilience within individuals on the journey to recovery, emphasizing the transformative potential inherent in the recovery process.

Myth 4: Addiction Only Affects Certain Demographics

Stereotypes about the demographics affected by addiction contribute to stigmatization. Chapter 14 examines how addiction transcends socioeconomic status, race, gender, and age, emphasizing its universality. Dispelling the myth of selectivity in the impact of addiction challenges preconceived notions, fostering a recognition that anyone, regardless of background, can be affected, and thus, deserves empathy, understanding, and support.

Myth 5: Treatment is Always Successful on the First Attempt

The expectation that treatment for addiction is always successful on the first attempt sets unrealistic standards. This chapter delves into the complexities of the recovery journey, acknowledging that relapses may occur and that the path to sustained recovery is often marked by setbacks and challenges. Dispelling the myth of immediate success cultivates a realistic understanding of the recovery process and the importance of ongoing support and resilience.

Myth 6: Addiction is a Reflection of Weak Character

Attributing addiction to weak character oversimplifies the intricate interplay of factors contributing to substance use disorders. Chapter 14 navigates the nuances of character and the multifaceted nature of addiction, emphasizing that it is not a moral failing but a complex health condition. Dispelling the myth of character judgement encourages a shift towards empathy, recognizing that individuals with addiction deserve understanding, support, and opportunities for recovery.

Myth 7: People with Addiction Don't Want to Get Better

Assumptions about the desires of individuals with addiction can perpetuate stigmatization. This chapter explores the ambivalence often experienced by those with substance use disorders, acknowledging the internal struggles they face. Dispelling the myth that individuals with addiction don't want to get better fosters a more compassionate understanding of the challenges inherent in seeking and sustaining recovery.

Media Portrayals and Stigmatization

The influence of media portrayals on stigmatization is a significant aspect of breaking the stigma. Chapter 14 scrutinizes how sensationalized depictions and stigmatizing language in media contribute to societal biases. By dispelling the myths perpetuated by media narratives, readers gain insights into the role of responsible communication in fostering a more accurate and empathetic public perception of addiction.

The Impact of Stigma on Mental Health

Stigma not only affects individuals with addiction but also has profound implications for mental health. This chapter examines the mental health consequences of stigmatization, including increased stress, shame, and reluctance to seek help. Dispelling myths becomes a means of mitigating the negative impact of stigma on mental well-being, encouraging open dialogue, and promoting a supportive environment for those affected by addiction.

Educational Initiatives: Fostering Understanding

Breaking the stigma involves educational initiatives aimed at fostering a deeper understanding of addiction. This chapter explores the role of education in dispelling myths, providing accurate information, and promoting awareness about the complexities of substance use disorders. By engaging in educational efforts, readers can contribute to challenging stereotypes and fostering a more informed and empathetic society.

Personal Narratives: Humanizing the Experience

Personal narratives play a pivotal role in humanizing the experience of addiction and dispelling myths. Chapter 14 examines the power of storytelling in sharing lived experiences, challenging stereotypes, and fostering empathy. By amplifying diverse voices and narratives, readers gain a more nuanced understanding of addiction, recognizing the resilience, challenges, and humanity within each individual on their journey to recovery.

Language Matters: Shaping Perspectives

The language used to describe addiction significantly shapes societal perspectives. This chapter delves into the impact of stigmatizing language and the importance of adopting person-first language that emphasizes the individual rather than the condition. By choosing language that respects the dignity of those with addiction, readers contribute to breaking down the linguistic barriers that perpetuate stigmatization.

Community Involvement: Building Supportive Networks

Breaking the stigma requires community involvement and the building of supportive networks. This chapter explores how communities can play a role in dispelling myths, challenging stigmatizing attitudes, and providing a supportive environment for individuals in recovery. By fostering community engagement, readers contribute to creating spaces where empathy, understanding, and compassion prevail over judgment.

Policy Advocacy: Addressing Structural Stigmatization

Structural stigmatization within policies can exacerbate societal biases. Chapter 14 examines the importance of policy advocacy in addressing systemic issues, challenging discriminatory practices, and promoting evidence-based approaches to addiction. By actively participating in policy initiatives, readers contribute to dismantling the structural barriers that perpetuate stigmatization.

Celebrating Recovery: A Positive Narrative

Shifting the narrative from stigmatization to celebration of recovery becomes a transformative aspect of breaking the stigma. This chapter explores how highlighting success stories, acknowledging achievements in recovery, and celebrating resilience contribute to a positive and hopeful narrative. By emphasizing the potential for growth and renewal, readers actively participate in reshaping societal perceptions of addiction.

Conclusion of Chapter 14:

Conclusion of Chapter 14: As we conclude our exploration of "Breaking the Stigma: Dispelling Myths," we stand at a crossroads—a pivotal moment where understanding, empathy, and action intersect. This chapter serves as a compelling reminder that addiction is not a moral failing or a choice but a complex health condition deserving of compassion and evidence-based support. By dismantling myths surrounding addiction, we pave the way for a more accurate and nuanced understanding of the challenges individuals face on their journey to recovery. Dispelling misconceptions about willpower, success on the first attempt, and the demographics affected by addiction fosters empathy and opens the door to more inclusive, supportive communities. The impact of stigmatization on mental health cannot be understated. As we break down the barriers of judgement and shame, we create space for individuals to seek help without fear of reproach. Educational initiatives, personal narratives, and mindful language choices become powerful tools in reshaping societal perspectives, challenging stereotypes, and fostering a culture of empathy. Community involvement and policy advocacy are crucial components of the journey to break the stigma. By actively participating in efforts that address systemic issues and promote evidence-based approaches, we contribute to the creation of environments that support rather than condemn those affected by addiction. As we celebrate recovery and highlight the resilience of individuals on their path to healing, we contribute to a positive and hopeful narrative. By emphasizing success stories, acknowledging achievements, and recognizing the humanity within each individual, we actively reshape the overarching societal perception of addiction. In concluding this chapter, we are reminded that breaking the stigma is not a solitary endeavour—it is a collective responsibility. Each reader, armed with knowledge and understanding, has the power to challenge stereotypes, foster empathy, and contribute to a society where individuals seeking recovery are met with support, understanding, and the recognition that their journey is one of strength, resilience, and hope.

Conclusion of Series 1: "Breaking Free: Overcoming the Grip of Drug Addiction"

As we draw the curtain on Series 1, "Breaking Free: Overcoming the Grip of Drug Addiction," we find ourselves at a juncture of reflection, understanding, and anticipation. This series has been a comprehensive exploration into the multifaceted dimensions of addiction—unmasking its complexities, deciphering its neurobiological intricacies, and delving into the societal impact that reverberates far beyond individual struggles.

The journey began with the foundational premise that breaking free from the chains of drug addiction is not only possible but a deeply transformative process. The title itself, "Breaking Free," serves as a beacon of hope, guiding readers through a terrain where resilience, knowledge, and support converge to illuminate the path to recovery.

In the initial chapters, we unmasked addiction—recognized the insidious nature of its grip and delved into the intricate web it weaves around individuals. The exploration of hidden triggers, the neurobiology of addiction, and the societal impact shed light on the pervasive reach of substance use disorders. We navigated the personal stories of unmasking, recognizing the diverse and often challenging journeys individuals undertake when facing addiction head-on.

The series unfolded like a roadmap, guiding readers through the terrain of addiction with compassion and empathy. From recognizing early signs to understanding the science behind addiction, each chapter served as a compass, offering insights, tools, and knowledge to empower individuals, families, and communities.

As we dissected the impact on cognitive function, we confronted the stark realities of how substance use can affect memory, decision-making, and emotional regulation. However, embedded within this exploration was the seed of hope—a recognition that the brain, with its remarkable neuroplasticity, has the potential for renewal, even in the aftermath of addiction.

Series 1 wasn't merely an academic endeavour; it was a call to action. It prompted readers to engage with the material, to reflect on their own beliefs and biases, and to consider how they might contribute to the destigmatization of addiction. Breaking down the myths surrounding addiction became not just a goal but a responsibility—one that requires collective efforts to reshape societal narratives and foster a more compassionate understanding.

The personal narratives shared throughout the series played a pivotal role in humanizing the experience of addiction. Real stories, with their highs and lows, successes and setbacks, served as a testament to the resilience of the human spirit. They underscored the importance of acknowledging that the journey to recovery is not linear but marked by growth, setbacks, and, above all, the determination to persevere.

As we explored the impact on cognitive function, delved into neuroplasticity, and broke down stigmas, the underlying theme remained consistent: recovery is a multifaceted process that extends beyond individual willpower. It requires understanding, support, and a holistic approach that considers the biological, psychological, and social dimensions of addiction.

The conclusion of Series 1 is not a finale but a transition— a bridge to what lies ahead. The seeds planted in understanding addiction, the exploration of cognitive function, and the dispelling of myths are poised to blossom in Series 2. This journey is a continuum, each series building upon the foundations laid by the preceding one.

As readers, you carry with you the insights gained from Series 1—an arsenal of knowledge and empathy to navigate the complexities of addiction. The stories shared, the neuroscientific principles explored, and the myths dispelled collectively serve as a compass for the road ahead. Armed with this understanding, you are not just passive consumers of information but active participants in the journey toward breaking free from the grip of drug addiction.

Series 1 closes, not with finality, but with the promise of continued exploration, growth, and transformation. The path to breaking free is ongoing, and Series 2 awaits, ready to delve deeper into the science, the stories, and the societal nuances that shape the landscape of addiction and recovery.

As we bid farewell to Series 1, let the knowledge gained be a catalyst for change—change in perspectives, change in actions, and, most importantly, change in the lives touched by the profound journey of breaking free from the grip of drug addiction.